ORTHOSTATIC TREMOR:
Am I the Only One?

JANE BAKER CONNER

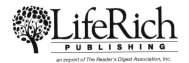

an imprint of The Reader's Digest Association, Inc.

LifeRich Publishing books may be ordered
through booksellers or by contacting:

LifeRich Publishing
1663 Liberty Drive
Bloomington, IN 47403
www.liferichpublishing.com
1 (888) 238-8637

ISBN: 978-1-4897-0044-5 (sc)
ISBN: 978-1-4897-0045-2 (e)

Printed in the United States of America.

LifeRich Publishing rev. date: 11/03/2013

Dedicated to: "Doris of Modesto",
my beacon of hope for the journey

Preface: Imagine having an ailment that no one can diagnose? Once named, it can't be cured.

And yet, if only one reader finds help and hope from my story, I will be ecstatic.

CHAPTER ONE:
"What in the Sam Hill?"

I T STARTS IN MY EARLY FIFTIES. AN INSURANCE agent, I find myself in the backyard of a favorite insured's home in Sausalito. Armed with notebook and Polaroid camera, I've come to update the renewal data. Now it's time to leave through the grassy steps, up the slope, through the gate. It was easy coming down, but suddenly my knees go weak and shaky, like they won't support me. My client is still at work, so I'm on my own. In desperation, I get down on all fours and claw my way up. Once safely back in my car, I ask myself "What just happened?" and answer "Jane, you really need to start Jazzercise or something to get your muscles stronger".

Then begins a period of new awareness of occasions when my legs fail me. When standing in a still position, they feel heavy and unsteady, as if I'm going to fall. Standing in a church memorial circle, we're singing when suddenly my legs start to shake; the 80-year-old lady next to me helps me to a chair. Why? "Probably just emotion." Standing in the corner of a party gathering, the shaking starts, and I lean against the wall. "Maybe reaction to alcohol." Standing in line at the BART station, I'm embarrassed that I can't stand in place for three or four minutes, so I ask the person behind me to hold my place in line while I go sit down. Now I'm pretending to be normal, but other people are vital to my being able to cope. Since the shaky legs also happen in line at the bank, the post office, and the supermarket, this is probably not psychological. It's time to get help.

I will spend ten years seeking answers. I will visit primary care physicians, neurologists, psychiatrists, physical therapists, gyms, and sports medicine, to no avail. No one has seen my symptoms before. Meanwhile, I try to hide the tremors at work and in social situations by sitting as much as possible. The church choir director lets me sit on a stool when it's time to stand. I even have one knee replaced, due to severe arthritis, thinking there might be some residual change. My wings are getting clipped; I turn down any invitations to stand and speak publicly.

All along, I've been sharing my frustration with a church friend, another Jane, who happens to have Essential Tremor, a shaking of the hands and/or head (yes-yes, no-no). Jane suggests that I try going to an Essential Tremor Support Group, just to hear how others cope. The Group turns out to be a light-hearted combination of various ages and stages of impairment, who meet monthly to share experiences, triumphs, and success with different (and sometimes new) medications. I leave the meetings feeling a little better about myself, although these folks all have different tremors than I do. Am I the only person on God's green earth that can walk but not stand still?

CHAPTER TWO: "Bingo!"

ONE SATURDAY, AT ET SUPPORT GROUP, the discussion turns to the doctors who've been helpful. My ears perk up at the mention of "Dr. Rosen", a neurologist in my HMO, who specializes in movement disorders. Yes, I'm still trying, so I make an appointment. It is the year 2000.

Dr. Rosen is a personable, animated redhead. She asks me to stand, and within five minutes, she has a diagnosis: Orthostatic Tremor, also known as "shaky leg syndrome". The condition is relatively rare. As of 1992, 28 cases have been reported. The cause is unknown. It is explained to me that somehow, there is less "insulation" or "layers of buffering" in the nerve wiring in my brain, so the circuitry allows impulses to pass through, down to my legs, causing severe contractions of the muscles of both legs, simultaneously. Many patients find it almost impossible to remain standing for more than 10-20 seconds, feel imbalanced, and need to sit down or lean against a wall for support. Despite the shakiness I feel inside, the tremor may not be visible on the outside. Remarkably, it disappears as soon as I take a step, sit, or lie down. For this reason, the disorder is typically misunderstood and often misdiagnosed as Parkinson's Disease by general physicians, as well as neurologists.

I remain standing; Dr. Rosen simply puts her hand on my legs and feels the trembling. Then she attaches surface electrodes connecting me to an electromyography (EMG) machine. Her diagnosis is confirmed by recordings of lower limb muscle tremor patterns at a frequency of 20 Hz (cycles per second). Like most OT patients, I don't have tremor of the hands, head, or voice common to Essential Tremor. The significant difference for diagnosis of OT is the high frequency of tremor (Essential Tremor range is 6-8 Hz).

Dr. Rosen explains more about orthostatic tremors. It affects men and women equally, usually in middle to late life. Family history is negative. It is a slow, progressive disorder with no known cure, but it's not life-threatening. There are a few medications that give marginal help to relieve the symptoms. We are going to use clonazepam (Klonopin) to begin.

Halleluiah! I don't like hearing all of this, but at least I have a name for my problem, at last. Now I can go on the Internet , specifically under "Primary Orthostatic Tremor", to search for new treatments and medicines. Did you catch that part about "no known cure"? That's why I will prowl OFTEN.

CHAPTER THREE:
"Coping" (or not?)

D R. ROSEN REFERS ME TO ANOTHER NEUROLOGIST in my HMO, "Dr. Karl", closer to home. He and I begin several years of trying different combinations and strengths of medicine, the last being Gabepentin (Neurontin).

Living with OT is challenging. At home, there are always walls to lean against or chairs to sit upon. I learn to take quick showers. My toes start to curl under ("hammer toes") from straining to grip the carpet, as if this could keep me upright. I get pretty good at chopping vegetables, deviling eggs, and mixing cookies sitting down.

Going on a cruise? Using the airport's wheelchair so works in the TSA lines. When the guide at Chichen

Itza stands us in the sweltering heat to lecture, I go to the rear, where I can still hear but keep moving. (I have since purchased a cane with a folding seat attached). For a couple of years, I lecture on cruises by teaching needlepoint on "at sea" days. I pass out hundreds of small coin or credit card purses, teaching how to stitch, thus offering entertainment and possibly a new skill— all do-able with a mike, a chart-easel, and a stool.

I admit to feeling panic in public—being caught in line somewhere like the bank with those thin ropes to stand between or meeting someone who stops me to chat. I choose to do shopping, bill paying, and banking by mail or computer. Using a cane in public explains part of my story.

I turn 65 and retire from 25 years of personal lines insurance, after 12 years of teaching elementary classes. Both of my careers have been teaching, really, just with different ages. Now I have the glorious gift of time, but admittedly, I lack the health and stamina to accomplish things of significance. I never planned on having my mobility challenged. The "Golden Years" were supposed to be time for grandchildren, for travel, for volunteering.

I feel the "wing clipping" again when I find myself not renewing play tickets, dropping out of church choir, and no longer able to keep my commitment to a favorite local women's chorale or special book groups. I face the fact I am consciously choosing social isolation because of OT. "Will you be able to navigate the entrance stairs at different homes?" "You know you're no longer responding to the medicine; do you still want to go—but in a wheel chair?"

This negative thinking is a spiral trap that is easy to fall into, but there is no comfort in staying there. When it happens, there are ways out. (I share suggestions in Chapter Five.)

CHAPTER FOUR:
A New Venture:
"Is DBS for You?"

O NE DAY, I'M PROWLING IN MY FAVORITE OT website when I come upon an article describing the use of DBS (Deep Brain Stimulation) to relieve the tremors of OT patients. It's a surgery being done successfully in Spain and Cincinnati. My friend Jane with ET has already had the DBS surgery and tells me it is marvelous. I can't wait to discuss this with Dr. Karl. Am I a candidate? I am 73 and in relatively good health. How could DBS help me? My tremors seem to be caused by "abnormal electrical messages generated by my brain. The DBS system delivers mild electrical therapy to block some of those messages. It may relieve the symptoms; however, it is not a cure."[1]

Dr. Karl explains that my HMO has had some success with DBS for Essential Tremor patients, but OT would be uncharted waters. A group of movement disorder specialists (neurologists and neurosurgeons) would have to deliberate on the efficacy of implanting DBS, after we furnish a number of tests, since I would be the first, at least in northern California. So we do EMG and video recordings, to be followed by CT scans (computer-aided tomography), MRIs (magnetic resonance imaging), and psycho-neurological tests (to rule out dementia). The time is November, 2011. It is fortuitous timing, as the medications are no longer effective.

While I'm waiting for my HMO's decision, it's worth inquiring around the Bay Area, so I call a couple of teaching hospitals. I learn that one, hence referred to as "Hope Hospital", is participating in a clinical research study evaluating an investigational device for Essential Tremor: a surgical procedure called deep brain stimulation. Have they tried DBS with Orthostatic Tremors? Yes, in January of 2011, a "Dr. Stanley" performed the first OT DBS surgery for patient "Doris of Modesto". I become acquainted with Dr. Stanley's clinical nurse and programmer whom I'll call "Angie". She says that Hope Hospital may be able to offer me surgery, if my HMO declines.

---

1   Your Medtronic Deep Brain Stimulation Therapy (Therapy-specific Patient Booklet, 2010, p.13

Eventually, with Doris' permission to contact her, obtained by Angie, I have the joy of speaking to Doris on the phone. Both the surgery and DBS programming are apparently successful. Doris can walk, drive, and stand in place for at least 25 minutes. In addition, she cares for a two-year-old great-grandson. I am incredulous to learn of her progress and achievements, almost a year after the surgery.

So just what is this DBS? Based on a discovery by a French surgeon in the 1980's, guided by CT scans and MRIs, a neurosurgical team implants a probe into the base of the brain, to stimulate the thalamus with high frequency electrical pulses. It has the same effect as the older technique of thalamotomy, without making a lesion (tissue permanently destroyed). It is possible to treat both sides of the brain at once, with only one neurostimulator implanted.

"The DBS system is implanted inside the body and includes 3 major parts:

1. <u>The lead</u> – The lead is a set of thin wires covered with a protective coating. It carries the therapy signal to the electrodes that deliver stimulation to the brain. Approximately 10 cm. (4 in.) of the lead is implanted in the brain. The rest of the lead (about 38 cm. or 15 in.) is implanted under the skin of the scalp.[2]

---

2   Your Medtronic Deep Brain Stimulation Therapy (Patient Therapy Guide), 2010, pp.24.

2. <u>The extension</u> – The extension is a set of thin wires covered with a protective coating that connects the lead to the neurostimulator. The extension is connected to the end of the lead, just behind the ear. The connection point between the lead and the extension is placed under the scalp. The remaining length of the extension is placed under the skin down the neck to the upper chest area and connects to the neurostimulator. There is one extension for each lead.

3. <u>The neurostimulator</u> –"The neurostimulator contains the power source of the DBS system. It generates and controls the therapy stimulation. The neurostimulator is implanted just under the skin in the upper chest area."[3]

In layman's terms, a small hole is drilled in the skull so a delicate wire with four tiny electrodes on the end is inserted deep in the thalamus, at the base of the brain. This may be repeated on the other side, the wires connected, and then passed down one side of the head and neck with an extension, to a pacemaker-like device implanted just below the collarbone, a battery. "To replace the battery, the doctor must replace the neurostimulator. This is a minor surgical procedure and is typically done as outpatient surgery, using a local anesthetic."[4]

---

3   P.25

4   P.38

The neurologist has a communicating battery-driven device, the shape of a TV remote control. When it is time to begin programming, he or she will put an antenna pad over the patient's shoulder and use a stylus, tapping variation of rate, pulse width, and amplitude. This initial setting is called Group A and can be programmed differently for Left Brain/Right Body and Right Brain/Left Body. During programming, the patient feels tingles of electricity in different places. If the change is uncomfortable or causes slurring in speech, it can be adjusted. The patient has a similar hand-held, external device and antenna, the size of a hefty cellphone, using two AAA batteries. This is placed against the chest to turn the system on or off or make stimulation adjustments in voltage, as tolerated. This is called a "patient programmer".

"The risks of DBS therapy include the risks of surgery and possible side effects or device complications. Implanting the brain stimulation system carries the same risks associated with any other brain surgery. Risks may include:

- Pain, inflammation, or swelling at the surgery sites
- Infection
- Headache
- Confusion or attention problems
- Bleeding inside the brain (stroke)

- Temporary or permanent neurologic complications
- Leakage of fluid surrounding the brain
- Seizures
- Paralysis, coma, or death
- Allergic response to implanted materials[5]

Possible side effects of DBS "may include:

- Tingling sensation (paresthesia)
- Temporary worsening of the patient's disease symptoms
- Speech problems like whispering (dysarthria) and trouble forming words (dysphasia)
- Vision problems (double vision)
- Dizziness or lightheadedness (disequilibrium)
- Facial and limb muscle weakness or partial paralysis (paresis)
- Movement problems or reduced coordination"[6]

Still very new therapy, there is NO GUARANTEE of improvement. The patient must commit initially six months of time and money to seek optimal DBS settings. DBS does not work in some patients because 1) the DBS system itself is not working properly, 2) the DBS settings

---

5   Your Medtronic Deep Brain Stimulation Therapy (Patient Therapy Guide), 2010, pp.31-32

6   Your Medtronic Deep Brain Stimulation Therapy (Therapy-specific Patient Booklet), 2010, pp.20-21

are not programmed properly, and 3) the electrodes are not in the best location.

I share this information with family and friends. I must admit the whole procedure is scary. I ask myself "What if something goes awry, and you come out of surgery like a vegetable?" My confidants may be thinking the same thing, but no one expresses the fear. The consensus is "Go for it!". For the quality of life offered, DBS is worth the risk. Now the wait begins.

CHAPTER FIVE:
"Nine Months to Go Before New Birth"

I CANNOT KNOW IT WILL TAKE 9 MONTHS FOR my HMO to approve my candidacy for surgery. I do remember it as a stressful time of anxiety and uncertainty. Am I making the right choice? Will DBS really work for me? I'm reminded by an old learning: "Faith and doubt cannot live in the same body." I can either lean on Trust that my God continues to care for me, or give in to worry that "just because it worked for Doris..." So I choose to think, "Yes, Doris is 10 years younger and yes, we have different brains; but we DO share the same Loving Maker."

How can I get through this time of of waiting? It

requires a time of self-talk, past the pessimism. My list of "how-to's" looks like this:

- Pray for patience.
- Make a list of gratitudes/positives in your life.
- Keep busy.
- Reach out to your social support.
- Get out of the house with short walks and drives.
- Escape with books.
- Exercise your brain with games.
- Increase your vocabulary with crossword puzzles, like the N.Y. Times.

And my Gratitudes:

- Faith to lean upon
- Hope in abundance
- My cheering squad of my family, friends, and church
- "Doris of Modesto"
- Cats (4) to offer companionship
- A brain that still works
- Awareness of others with deeper challenges
- Glasses to read and see details
- The healing power of sleep
- Life itself—time to find meaning in struggle

In late summer of 2011, the HMO approves DBS for me. My neurologist assures me that the chosen neurosurgeon," Dr. Gray", is not just very competent, "He is phenomenal". In our consultation, Dr. Gray prefers two sessions of surgery, for greater accuracy in lead placement. The first one (left side of my brain) is scheduled for early August.

I arrive at the hospital promptly at 6 A.M. Dr. Gray is ready, together with a "Dr. Martin", standing beside him. His assistant shaves the left side of my head. Off goes the hair; on goes a metal frame to keep my head from moving and assist in lead placement. A local anesthetic is used, because the frame is actually screwed in place.

Off to the OR. The surgical team has already reviewed my MRI and CT scans to guide the optimal placement of the lead. Now it's time to "numb my scalp before creating a small hole in the skull for the lead to pass through. Later in the surgery, the lead will be locked in place on the outside of the skull with a specially designed cap (which also covers the hole)."[7]

The only memory I have of the OR is humorous, if embarrassing. I am lightly sedated. The team is testing areas of the brain by sending currents of tingle to parts of me, so I can respond "elbow", "fingertip", "jawbone". Suddenly I blurt out, "If you guys aren't careful, we're going to get a climax here." I hear all these men roaring. Someone says, "We should invite Jane back tomorrow

---

7   Your Medtronic Deep Brain Stimulation Therapy (Patient Therapy Guide), 2010, p.41

for more laughs." Normally, I would be mortified to have said such a thing, but I've since been told that these impromptu moments add fun to the long day of proper protocol.

The surgery goes well, the stimulation target is located, and the lead is passed into my brain. As could be expected, I have nausea in recovery but do well after that, staying in the hospital just two days after surgery. I'm grateful for the pain medicine given for the headaches which do come, once I'm home. I am given my very own Medtronic patient programmer, video, and guidebooks to help me understand DBS, a trademark of Medtronic, Inc. I wish I had been given this information before the surgery.

Two weeks later, it's time to return for the right side of my head (right brain controls the left side of my body). The only disconcerting thing is the absence of Dr. Gray. I'm told "He's ill; Dr. Martin will be in charge." I already know the drill for the hair shaving and head frame. The surgery has to be longer this time, because it involves inserting the right lead, connecting with the left lead. Then extensions go behind the right ear, along the neck, to join the neurostimulator newly implanted just below the collar bone in the chest. All goes as planned. I'm released, with the next procedure to be removing the sutures. It takes time for the brain swelling to diminish, about four weeks. The "main event" will be turning the DBS *on*, followed by the first programming, in September. I'm so excited that I can hardly sleep the night before.

This special appointment involves going to Sacramento. I am to see a neurologist who was one of the original committee approving the surgery. He requested doing the first programming for me. We spend over an hour together. Using his clinician programmer, "Dr. Arthur" methodically checks each contact, with me telling him what sensation I feel and where I feel it. He asks me to stand from time to time, walk a bit, and talk, so he can check any change in speech. I'm surprised to hear myself instantly slurring some words as if intoxicated; but he makes adjustments and says this will dissipate. I still have tremors when standing in place, but it's going to take time for my brain to process the new stimulation. So we go home and wait.

CHAPTER SIX:
"Are We There Yet?"

THE FALL HAPPENS, REGARDLESS. MY FAMILY AND friends are faithfully encouraging. There are a handful of "glorious days" when I'm out and about feeling terrific, almost tremor-free. I can drive, shop, and go to my appointments alone. I begin seeing my neurologist in Walnut Creek, Dr. Karl, for the fine tuning of my settings, about twice a week. I seem to be most comfortable with low voltage of 1.5 – 1.6. One time, Dr. Karl turns me up to 1.7. Once home, I can't make it out of the car, which is scary. We head back to the doctor immediately, as I haven't yet been taught how to make any setting adjustment by myself. That day comes, along with the day Dr. Karl determines that the initial setting in September throws the energy to my mouth/speech areas. Every time he tries to increase the voltage of the lower electrodes (left or right), my speech falls apart, like one sounds after Novocain at the dentist. My tongue and lips feel puffy. It's work to form words correctly. Dr. Karl decides to change the initial settings.

I receive a postcard from IETF (International Essential Tremor Foundation, PO Box 14005, Lenexa, KS 66285-4005, phone (888) 387-3667, essentialtremor. org) inviting me to a Support Group Meeting featuring a "Hope Hospital" neurosurgeon. The topic? "Surgical Treatments for Essential Tremor". The place? Same location I went to in the past. I RSVP with the leader, whom I remember.

It feels good to be back. One gentleman named "Joe" has had a successful DBS implant for his Essential Tremor, and he demonstrates "now" and "then". He stands before us, perfectly still, with no tremor. Then he takes out his patient programmer, puts it over his chest, and switches the battery off. Immediately, his left hand flies up and all over the place. Joe quips, "You can see why I was popular at parties, to shake the cocktails." It is a dramatic demonstration of "before" and "after" DBS. The speaker was Joe's neurosurgeon.

Weeks pass. Dr. Karl diligently tries various settings over twenty-some appointments between September, 2011 and March, 2012. There's a setback in November due to an attack of gout; the pain and medication don't help with standing or walking. Home Health comes. A wheelchair is rented to give me more independence in mobility. The holidays are a bit depressing, but cards and calls lift my spirits. Frustrated and worried, I decide to ask my HMO to authorize my going to Hope Hospital for a second opinion, in hopes of "the right settings". Dr. Karl requests permission. It comes for the March 30th consultation.

Knowing of the second opinion request, there is a flurry of attention from my HMO neurology. I'm called and asked to return to Sacramento, where Dr. Arthur tries "constant current" settings for the first time (vs. "constant voltage"), but there's no change. Then the surgeon's Physician Assistant requests an updating CT scan, which happens on February 27th. When I call for the results, he advises "Just don't let anything press against your neck, as the wire is very close to the surface". Looking back, it seems this is a prime time for the surgeon to study the CT scan and address any problems. However, nothing changes for me.

March 30, 2012 finally arrives. I meet with a team of Hope Hospital neurologists. They test each and every electrode, create a new "C" program, and request my HMO to send copy of the February 27th CT scan. Early in May, the neurologist calls with shocking news. Both a neurosurgeon, "Dr. Stanley" and the neurologists have reviewed the scan. I am told "The leads are not placed properly. Further programming will not be fruitful".

I need a new authorization to discuss this with Dr. Stanley on July 11th. It seems that doing nothing means NO CHANCE for change.

My initial reaction to this news is frustration, even anger. I have wasted seven months of re-programming trips, with no significant improvement, because the DBS system isn't set up correctly. In fact, if I hadn't gone to Hope in March, I would still be trekking to Dr. Karl on a hopeless quest, a total waste of his and my time, as well as the HMO's resources. I can't help thinking "Why didn't MY surgeon see the problem from the same CT scan?" Now I'm in the uncomfortable position of having to ask him for permission to see another surgeon outside the system, to fix the problem.

It turns out that both surgeons are acquainted and easily communicate and agree on their findings. Leads may migrate after the implant, there may be "brain shift" due to the necessary introduction of air at time of surgery, or there may be mal-positioning originally because of other factors. Placement is such a delicate art, with exact "targets" unknown, all part of a relatively new procedure.

At any rate, I do get to meet "Dr. Stanley" on July 11th. There is a serendipity in this consultation. A stunning young woman, with lovely blond hair up in a bun, joins us. She is "Dr. Reynolds", and she has a Fellowship with Dr. Stanley. In layman's terms, this means she shadows Dr. Stanley all day, learning neurosurgery "in the trenches". Best of all, she happens to have earned her degree from Indiana University, which is also my alma mater. We reminisce about Hoosier favorites—the autumnal beauty of Brown County, historic Spring Mill, and the famous biscuits of "Nashville House".

The three of us review my history. Dr. Stanley records that I am in a wheelchair, but I can get up and walk when I get started from a standing position. I am at significant risk of falling when turning. I'm unable to stand up and be still for more than 30 seconds, which impacts my ability to do activities outside the home.

Dr. Stanley explains the DBS lead revision process. The new lead will be put beside the old one, and then the old lead is removed. A new MRI is required for a closer look at the left lead, which may not need revision. The MRI scan will be done with the hospital's low-energy protocol. Usually a 3 mm. "off prime location" is the deciding factor.

The surgery will take 3-5 hours. The risks are 1-3% for stroke and 3% for infection. Typically, a patient stays 2-3 days in the hospital. Three weeks later, I am to return to Angie for staple removal and first programming. Dr. Stanley hopes I can stay with Hope Hospital Movement Disorder Specialists as long as the HMO allows, probably six months. He is available for surgery in August or October. Yes, Dr. Reynolds will be there in the OR. He believes my HMO will say "yes".

We discuss extensively the use of DBS for orthostatic

tremor. Dr. Stanley cautions about depending on Internet advice, as it only touts the successes. It is unknown how many DBS efforts with OT have failed. We do know there are less than 5 success cases reported in the world literature, not counting the one surgery performed a year ago at Hope Hospital. He gives me a 50% chance of my being able to benefit from DBS for orthostatic tremor, based on the very small numbers that have been done. (I think to myself "but the odds were always 50-50".)

I ask if there is a "best target" for me. No, it is not known for the treatment of OT, but Dr. Stanley's group and others have generally placed leads in the same thalamic location as used for other tremor, such as essential tremor. I ask "Is that what you did for 'Doris of Modesto'?" "Yes", he replies. I say "Then that's what I want for me".

Having now met Dr. Stanley for the first time, I find him very professional, personable, and humble. I am so comfortable and confident with him that this is an easy decision. Now I must tell my HMO that I want Dr. Stanley to do the repositioning and all the reasons why, as they are expecting my return to them.

CHAPTER SEVEN:
"A Moment of "Truth"

INITIALLY, THE TASK SEEMS FORMIDABLE, BECAUSE my HMO contract requires me to get all of my medical care from its providers, when there is a competent doctor available. Obviously, I prefer to have the repositioning surgery done by Dr. Stanley because he has performed thousands of DBS surgeries and most importantly, tackled OT specifically and successfully with "Doris of Modesto". I am living proof that my implant needs correction. I have only one brain to risk, yet again. I worked diligently with the HMO's neurology for seven months of re-programming, to no avail.

How to start? It seems I need an advocate to navigate the system. I begin by calling my HMO Member Services for the telephone number for Contra Costa County

Senior Aging Information and Assistance. The person listens patiently and pleasantly, quickly grasping the issue. He refers me to HICAP (1-800-510-2020, Health Insurance Counseling Assistance Program) to explain my HMO and Medicare benefits.

Because I am over 60 and live in Contra Costa County, I am eligible for a free 30 minutes' consultation with an attorney (Walnut Creek Senior Center (925) 943-5851. The Law Center at (866) 543-8017 offers assistance in obtaining free or sliding scale legal representation.

The HICAP gentleman is very knowledgeable and helpful. I have two options:

1) I have to file a referral request with my HMO to go outside the system for repositioning surgery. The letter must be overwhelmingly convincing—simple, direct, and without anger. If my request is denied, it can always be appealed.

2) Return to original Medicare - 80/20 payments (Open Enrollment is coming Oct. 15 to Dec. 7th.) and choose a Medicare Drug Plan. The upside is being able to choose any doctor without needing authorization. The downside is having to wait until after Jan. 1, 2013 (effective date) for possible surgery.

I turn to my friends for advice about the referral request letter. One person suggests having a video made, so I can tell my story straight from the wheelchair. It is not comfortable to be in an adversarial position with my HMO. Actually, I have many positive relationships with my doctors over the years. I do not want to burn any bridges. However, I am determined in my quest, with no intention of suing to get my way. The letter must have "some teeth in it". So the last words evolve "I hope to negotiate with you before I turn this over to my attorney".

It takes a week to write my so-carefully-worded request to the Member Case Resolution Center. On July 11th, I receive a phone call from the Senior Case Manager to confirm receipt and that my concerns are valid. He clarified that normally, this kind of letter would come AFTER the HMO surgeon files a referral to Outside Services, passes through the Chief of Neurology, then the Committee, and is denied. I respond that it is awkward for me to be confrontational with Dr. Martin. I say, "May I ask for an hour to think about it, and call back?" In that time, I decide it would probably work out better to stay in the systems' parameters and go through the process with Dr. Martin. So I ask to withdraw my letter for the time being.

The toughest part will be addressing Dr. Martin, who has offered and expects to do the repositioning surgery. Here is part of the first E-mail to him to explain my feelings. "This is very hard for me to say to you. You have always been so caring. My only grievance is that after you ordered the updating CT in February, you had the chance to see problems and make corrections. You didn't act; Dr. Stanley did. Now 4 months have passed; I am in the same dilemma". He answers that he did not order the CT scan or even know about it. He only heard about this after it went full circle, also learning that Dr. Stanley wanted to revise both electrodes. Then Dr. Martin analyzed the CT scan, calculating all the numbers in detail. He determined that only the right brain electrodes' position needed to be revised. Apparently, Dr. Stanley agrees with him. Dr. Martin also tells me he has no problem with my going to Dr. Stanley—that I should do whatever makes me feel most comfortable. Needless to say, this answer gives me so much relief.

Then begins a series of back-and-forth E-mails in which I ask Dr. Martin to *initiate the process*. His answer dumfounds me, as he says he will be glad to approve it if something comes his way. Ahh, the gentle art of communication… In all fairness, my hunch is that surgeons don't usually get involved with the paperwork of referrals. This turns out to be merely a hiccup along the way, as Dr. Martin then goes to "Samantha", Ombudsman Mediator in his building to ask her to assist me.

On July 7th, Samantha calls me, listens, and understands. The only problem is that she's never done this process before, but she is willing to try, after she researches. I share what I have learned so far and from whom. It's a good thing I have the twelve years of teaching experience to hone my patience.

Lo and behold, on August 3rd, Samantha calls to say that the Head of the Department has shown her the paper approving Hope Hospital surgery. It is dated July 16th. I am disappointed that no one called or wrote to ME, but at least I crossed a huge hurdle. I stop and wonder how much of a role Samantha played in all this. At least she will know the process next time.

I now have permission to call Hope and schedule a date with Dr. Stanley. Of course, by now the August surgery opening is already taken, but my name can be listed for October. In the meantime, I have the special MRI scan and blood work done.

In late September, there is a pre-op appointment in the office that is very significant. It is to review pre-op reading scales (detailed testing of all electrodes). In addition, the neurologists make videos of my walking with my existing DBS turned "on" and "off". They attach surface electrodes connected to and EMG machine, and record my tremors "on" and "off". With "off", the tremors are formidable when I am standing. They look like high Richter scale earthquakes on the screen. This tells all of us that even with one lead in the wrong place; I <u>still have benefit from the DBS system as a whole.</u> This is huge encouragement for any OT-DBS candidate.

This chapter had a special urgency for me to write, in the hopes that it may assist others in wending their way through possible red tape and bureaucracy. There was no "how to" in print for me. I am so grateful to all the encouragement and advice given in my pursuit, so I am happy to share what worked for me. Hopefully, as the best parts of Obamacare are implemented, my suggestions will become obsolete.

CHAPTER EIGHT:
"It Takes a Village to the Rescue"

THE DAY OF MY SURGERY, IT IS A JOY TO SEE BOTH Doctors Stanley and Reynolds ready for me—no last minute substitutions. Only the right brain electrodes will be moved. All goes well, with two events remembered. Near the end of the time, I recalled hearing Doctor Reynolds' voice above my head, repeating Dr. Stanley's instructions on "how to close". It seems that he is actually letting her have the experience. Then a third doctor leans in very close to my face, asking how I feel. My first response is "Oh, my, you have beautiful eyes". (We meet later, and his eyes ARE a very special blue.)

Some differences this time are no nausea, hallucinations, or headaches afterward. The only pain I feel is a sore throat, later attributed to the fact I coughed when I was in the head brace. They had to use suction aggressively so they could continue. After recovery, I feel euphoria—so amazingly good that I insist on calling family and friends myself.

I am released the third day, taken by ambulance to a skilled nursing facility in Concord. However, I have a seizure in the ambulance. This is not too unusual for a person who just had brain surgery. The staff can accept me until ... I get inside and start the admitting process, not knowing anything has happened. I am chatting away, when I black out with another seizure. Two seizures are more than the nursing facility can handle, so the decision is made to transport me to John Muir Hospital in Walnut Creek. The ER Doctors do an EKG and lab tests. They suspect heart damage from a silent heart attack, as the EKG is not satisfactory, and there are "markers on the blood". The next day, I am transported back to Hope Hospital for cardiology attention. Meanwhile, my HMO Primary Care doctor, "Dr. Wren", has been alerted. She steps up to the plate and orders a cardiology appointment for my eventual return to the East Bay.

In San Francisco, I am examined daily by the Neurology and Cardiology teams. My blood looks better each day. It seems less urgent that more invasive tests for blockage be done just now. One hurdle at a time; getting the brain healed is top priority for me. Athough the doctors propose doing a heart workup, the ambulance for Walnut Creek arrives. Just a week later, I do see the HMO cardiologist who prescribes beta-blockers and anti-seizure medication. She also orders a new EKG for the future.

Two weeks after the surgery, I return to Hope's Neurology to see Angie for my first programming. It takes over an hour as she methodically tests each electrode and records the results in term of my ability to stand, take steps, and speak. She send me home "turned on" in the best combination, and I have homework. I am to take the voltage of the right brain up one notch daily, i.e. 1.5 to 1.6 to 1.7, as long as it's comfortable. The first steps are easy, all the way to 2.0, but when I tried to go from 2.1 to 2.2, my speech is slurred and walking is wobbly. Angie says it is alright to stay put at 2.0 until our next visit.

In November, my HMO sends home nursing aids to my house. An RN, a physical therapist, and a social worker each come on different days. They routinely check my vital signs. This is how I learn my heart rate is consistently in the low forties, no matter what I do in movement. The therapist wonders if I even should be exercising. She calls my Dr. Wren, who suggests we cut the beta-blocker meds in half to get my heart pumping. I do feel better and have more energy. By the end of November, I get permission to stop taking the beta-blocker completely, so I can participate in my HMO's on-site physical therapy.

Dr. Wren rescues me still another time when I have serious choking, trying to swallow the huge anti-seizure pill, to the point of calling 911. The pills shouldn't be cut in half, so she orders a liquid form instead—problem solved.

Just before Thanksgiving, it is time to see Angie. She updates the records with new testing. This time she sets up group A, B, C, and D with varying contacts, voltage, pulse width, and frequency. Group A becomes my default group, the familiar one to go to if the others aren't working for me. I am to keep a daily journal, recording what happens. Since both sides are set at the same starting voltage, I get to experiment with both Right and Left, alternating the increase a notch, i.e. right up to 1.6, next day left up to 1.6, next day right up to 1.7, next day left up to 1.7. I will return to Angie in six weeks. Now this gives me options—settings to try on my own. This begins our new pattern of working together.

In January, I discover a "Best Day" setting in the company of my brother-in-law Don, visiting from Florida. I feel really good, confidently moving to the deck to sit in the sun, walking to his car to go to lunch, then inside the restaurant—all without my transport chair. So now I have a good Group C at 2.1 and 1.9.

My HMO Physical Therapist, " Veronica", has specialized in Neurological challenges. One of the valuable tips she gives me in the beginning is how to stand and sit gracefully. It has to do with basic body mechanics: get knees over toes, take a small bow, and then rise or sit. She explains that a person's head weighs about as much as a bowling ball. Instead of thinking "I must hold my head up as good posture", it seems making the little dip with the head does line up the body correctly to follow through gracefully. I learn to sit smoothly, without plopping. I stand correctly by positioning the knees apart over the toes, making the bow, and pushing off. Of course, it's all easier in a chair with arms.

Veronica invites me to a small weekly group of 5 or 6 patients in the gym setting, where I use the parallel bars, bicycle, and balance board. In a one-to-one consult, she suggests my "powering through the tremors", leaning against the wall. The idea is to build endurance. I can stand twenty minutes in her office. So I decide to try for 30 minutes at home in the kitchen with ear buds and a CD of the church choir's gospel-rock. This works for me, because: 1) I enjoy it and 2) I can do all my exercises upright without fear of falling. Another time, she suggests a 26" high stool for the kitchen counter. This way, I can see when the sauce has thickened, be close to the sink for chopping food, and be up higher to wash dishes. Her intent is to get me up doing something more practical than leaning against the wall.

In March, I am trying out a new group A setting and stumble up and down the voltage scale to find speech resolved at 2.0 and 2.0. This is exciting because it means Angie and I now have <u>two</u> comfortable settings, first in C and now A. We must be getting closer! I am beginning to see, in a rudimentary fashion, how Angie programs, trying and then eliminating that which doesn't work, modifying and re-offering that which <u>could.</u>

It is important for me to include this chapter illustrating how the referring HMO, the Hope Hospital Neurology staff, Angie, Doctor Wren, and Veronica have interacted so efficiently. In the beginning, I never dreamed that I would get in situations where I would need ALL of them to care for me, nor how much I would benefit from the overlapping of their services. This is the best of medicine, where the two providers are skillfully communicating in the patient's behalf. It has been an interesting journey to bring me to this awareness. No longer do I feel in an adversarial position with my HMO. They have been exceedingly patient and generous with me, allowing time to explore the unknown.

CHAPTER NINE:
"Success Story Number Five"

I T IS LATE MAY, 2013, AND I HAVE CABIN FEVER. It seems like the right time to try to meet "Doris of Modesto" in person, after two years of relating by telephone, mail, and E-mail. Modesto, being in the Central Valley, will be heating up soon for the summer. So I call her, and yes, she'll be home Saturday. It's fortuitous that we're to meet soon, as she's scheduled for knee replacement surgery in a few days.

My friend drives us to Doris' home. She comes out to the car, and her voice is just like on the phone—calm, collected, and comforting. She has twinkly eyes and is warm in her welcome. Her husband is at the door, showing us in.

The living room is cozy and filled with Doris' collections—plates, tea cups, and small dolls on the shelf, representing her ten siblings. There are picture frames of family galore—two sons, three grandsons and one great-grandson. The latter just turned three and has been cared for in this home while his daddy serves in Kuwait and his mother attends beauty school. Doris is around 65 and fully capable of that labor of love. In addition, she looks after elderly ladies near-by, on a daily basis, relating to them as a daughter.

Doris and I get caught up on our lives and progress. She can stand twenty minutes now and gets through most of her chores. She explains to me how this works. For example, she may be outside gardening when a neighbor walks by. Doris is able to stand chatting until she feels the tremors starting. Then she may say "Sorry, my time is up" and goes back inside. She rests a bit, and then she's able to do something else.

Doris seems cheerful and content with her life. She looks healthy, and I tell her how pretty her curly hair looks in a saucy pony tail. Doris looks younger than her years, probably because of her positive attitude. She is very practical and down-to-earth.

We talk of how when the phone rings, both of our families know of the "Doris and Jane" relationship; it's super special if either Doris or Jane is calling. We have our very own ups and downs to share because of the uniqueness of our orthostatic tremors and the DBS surgeries. I tell Doris how grateful I am to no longer feel like "the only one", since she has been down the same road, even before me. She is the only person I know who feels the same unsteadiness and uncertainty as I do, yet she never wavers in her assurance "It will all get better for us". Best of all, I can tell our "mutual admiration society" is to continue, because our affection and trust are very real. We take pictures and leave. Such a sweet lady—

CHAPTER TEN:
"Jane Wraps It Up, Still Learning"

A FTER THE LAST BRAIN SURGERY, I AM IN RECOVERY and suddenly inspired to write a book. I feel so very good, so hopeful, and so grateful that I feel almost compelled to write about my experience. In awhile, I am writing every day. In my Christmas cards, I add "When I'm 80% well, I'm going to write a book. Watch for AM I the ONLY ONE?" (as if I needed some measure of progress towards 100% or perfection).

Today, I see that was an unrealistic expectation, with or without tremors! I have been told many times that DBS is not a cure. It is intended to relieve the tremor symptoms. To be fair, I cannot discount the long way I have come. Once I no longer responded to medication, the decision to try for Deep Brain Stimulation surgery was the right choice for me. It turned out to offer much more quality of life than I had before, even when the electrodes were not in optimal position.

Now I feel an urgency to end the book, in order to get the word out. It took me ten years to find a diagnosis of orthostatic tremor; there must be others still seeking. I spent another ten years learning techniques of coping and exploring different drugs; others can benefit from my journey. Then Deep Brain Stimulation surgery came on the scene, bringing risks but also relief. I hope the reader will find some answers in my story. Lastly, because my HMO's implants weren't functioning correctly, I sought to go outside the system for re-positioning. There was no manual to teach me that process, so I wrote my own. I ended up teaching others. Ultimately, I benefitted hugely from *both* sides' care for me.

Now there is the gradual process of re-entering "real life" again. It involves more exercise and learning to embrace the challenges of new experiences and environments, always within the parameters of safety. I already know that when I'm patient with myself, I can make progress. That progress will happen faster with a positive attitude.

And what about all the superb human beings I've met along the way? I can't begin to name all of them, but you know who you are—my special family and friends—the cheering squad who sent loving prayers and encouragement all along , and of course, the wonderful medical community who did "the hard stuff" so skillfully. Interwoven throughout my journey is the enormous Peace of God's presence. It gives me personal satisfaction to humbly offer my memoirs, reaching out and giving back.

AUTHOR'S NOTE:

To preserve anonymity, I have used pseudonyms
for all medical persons and institutions.

It is a privilege to use quotes from the Medtronic, Inc. ©
patient materials "Your Medtronic Deep Brain
Stimulation Therapy" 2010 with the permission of
Medtronic, Inc. © 2010.

AUTHOR'S BIO

Jane Baker Conner was reared in Decatur, IL. She graduated summa cum laude 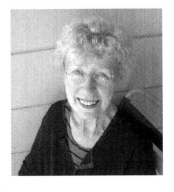 from Indiana University in 1960. Jane taught a variety of grades in elementary education for 12 years, then spending 25 years as a personal lines insurance agent. Mother of two, grandmother of five, Jane lives in Walnut Creek, CA with her four cats.

Made in the USA
San Bernardino, CA
30 March 2019